How to Use This Book

This book is intended to provide parents with an easy res[...] oils while providing children with a fun and interactive w[...] Read the pages with your children and keep oils close s[...] learning. Test the recommended techniques while reading. Keep this book close as a reference guide when you need to use oils on your children, and track your usage in the back pages so you know what works best for your kids. Most of all, have fun learning and teaching your child about the possibilities that are open to you in the world of essentail oils.

Additional Information

Children should use essential oils under the supervision of an adult.

Most essentail oils should be diluted with a carrier oil for use on children. Carrier oils are typically vegetable oils, such as olive oil, almond oil, or Young Living's V-6™ massage oil. Young Living's KidScents® Lotion or Lavender Hand & Body Lotion also work well as carriers. Make sure your carrier is organic so you're not rubbing pesticides and other synthetic chemicals into your children's skin.

For more extensive information about Essential oils and their properties, consult the Essential Oils Desk Reference from Essential Science Publishing.

Statements in this book have not been evaluated by the Food and Drug Administration. Statements/products in this book are not intended to diagnose, treat, cure, or prevent any disease. This book is for entertainment purposes only.

This book belongs to:

_____

Written and Illustrated by Amy J. Oler

Edited by Christopher B. Oler

Text and illustrations ©2009 Amy J. Oler. All rights reserved. No part of this book may be used or reproduced in any manner whatsoever without written permission of the publisher. The stories, characters, and/or incidents in this publication are entirely fictional. ISBN: 978-1492155713

I'm Brad and this is my sister Lisa. We're learning to use essential oils in our house.

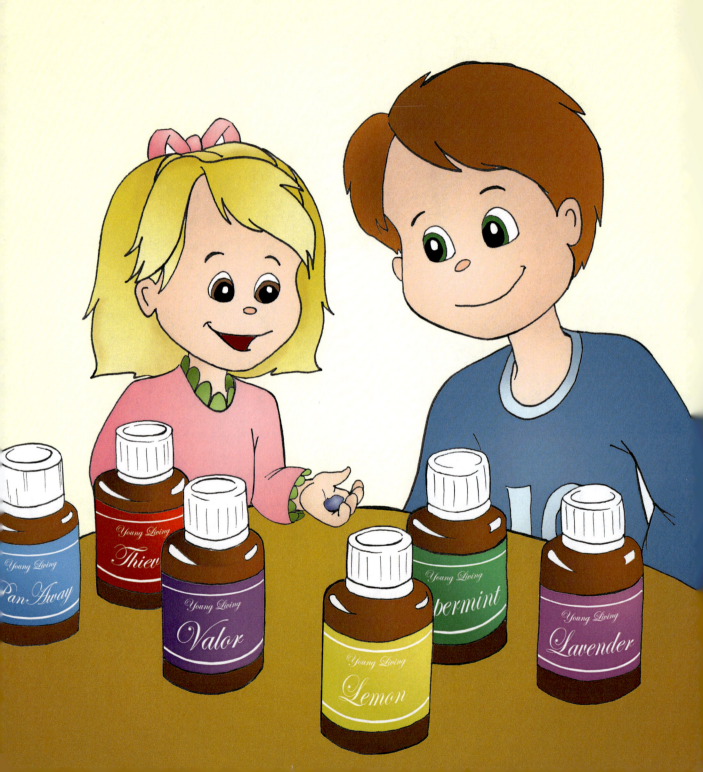

Overview of Essential Oils

What are they? Essential oils are distilled from flowers, trees, roots, bushes, and seeds; they can also be cold-pressed from fruit rinds.

Are they similar to the cooking oils in my kitchen? Essential oils differ from vegetable oils (ie, corn, olive, canola) in that they are not greasy, and if properly made, do not become rancid over time.

Why can Young Living oils sometimes cost more than other brands? Essential oils must be properly made in order to have therapeutic value. Many lower-cost oils are produced quickly by cheap methods, compromising purity and often creating toxicity. Make sure you know the history and integrity behind the company producing your oils. Young Living has a rich history of producing high-quality oils.

How long have people been using essential oils? Essential oils are the ancient medicines of mankind. Usage has been recorded as far back as 4500 BC. They were rediscovered in the 20th century, and have been studied in modern times since the 1930s.

Testimonials From Users

Duncan came to me with a look of misery on his face and said he had a stomach ache and it was bad ... I thought, "Oh yeah! A chance to try another oil!" He didn't know what caused it, but I put a drop of Di-Gize® in a glass of water and had him drink it, and rubbed a drop over his belly button. Literally, about 1½ minutes later, he announced it didn't hurt at all anymore. How in the *world*!?

I'm new to oils and every time I try them, it seems like magic. I hate to say it, but this is actually fun and amazing. I thought my kids would roll their eyes every time mom reached for the oils, but *they* are feeling first hand how they work and are converts themselves. God has really been blessing us at every turn in our lives. Discovering these oils by hearing the other moms at church talk about them has been the latest blessing. I would not have been open minded enough to try them had I not heard from them first how the oils have worked for their families.
—Mia Overton

I sustained a slightly fractured, very badly sprained ankle. The pain was so intense I laid on the couch and cried. I was unable to put any weight on it. My sons helped me alternate ice and the Young Living essential oils of Valor®, lavender, PanAway®, thyme, basil, marjoram, cypress, wintergreen, Aroma Siez®, grapefruit, lemongrass, and peppermint. With the help of my sons, I got into bed after three rounds each of ice and oils on my ankle. During the night I broke into a "healing sweat." The next morning (expecting to order crutches), I gently tested my feet on the floor. To my total amazement, I walked! I continued applying the oils several times a day for the next few days and less often afterwards. I walked with a slight limp, and two days later my walk was perfectly normal!

This is one of many positive outcomes I have had in eleven years of using Young Living essential oils—which point to the efficacy, quality, and purity of these extraordinary products. I stand firm in my conviction there are **no better essential oils in the world!**
—Jill Taylor

Essential oils are medicines made from plants like the flowers and leaves in my back yard.

Some are made from fruits, like lemons or oranges.

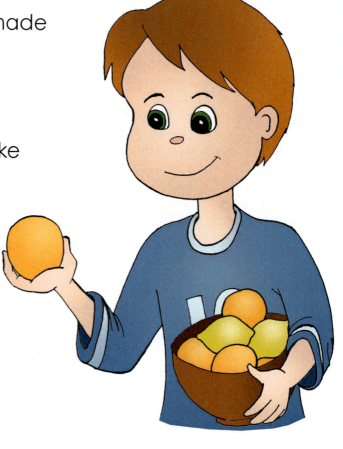

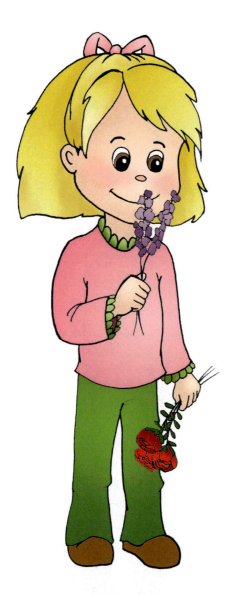

The special liquid is pulled out of the plant and put into bottles so it's easy for my family to use.

How to Use Essential Oils

How do I use them? Essential oils can be applied topically, taken internally, or used aromatically. Young Living's oils absorb quickly through the skin. They can be mixed with water for drinking, cooked with, or taken in capsules. Many of Young Living's nutritional supplements contain essential oils, which have been shown to increase absorbancy and effectiveness. Diffusing or breathing essential oils is an easy way to get them into the body, and can be especially useful for behavioral or emotional support.

What is a diffuser? A diffuser is a machine that distributes essential oils into the air. Diffusing can be an effective way to cleanse household air or dissipate a scent into a room. Effective diffusers have a high air saturation rate. Effective diffuser models can be found on the Young Living Web site.

Testimonials From Users

My daughter, Courtney, had chronic croup cough every winter and was borderline asthmatic. Her medications were albuteral through a breathing machine, and really strong antibiotics and cough medicines. Since nothing was working for her, the doctor then wanted to switch her meds to the "highest dosage"—the side effect was heart palpatations! My husband and I did not want this. That winter, when Courtney was 4 years old, my sister-in-law did a Raindrop Treatment on me. Our dog, Koda, was limping from stepping into a hole. Anna applied peppermint oil on Koda and he stopped limping! After seeing all this, Courtney was curious and wanted oils on her too. So, we put the Young Living peppermint oil all over her toes and the bottoms of her feet. She was fast asleep in 15 minutes and the next morning came running into our bedroom saying "Mommy, Daddy, I can breathe, I can breathe!" This was when we started using the oils regularly on Courtney and her baby sister, Megan. Courtney is now 6 years old and no longer has chronic croup cough and is off all her medications. Needless to say, she loves the oils because we no longer have to make her swallow medications. That is the best part, that my daughter does not have to gag down medicine anymore.
—*Jennifer DeSantis*

August will mark 2 years since I started the oils and I have many incredible stories. We just had our 7th child, my first oil baby, 5 weeks ago and I would *never ever* leave home without my oils. This stuff works better than *anything* the pharmacies or stores have, not even considering it is natural for the body—so no side effects! People don't understand what they're missing. Not only does it make us SUPER MOM to our own kids, but when we've got our oils with us, we go along through our day and are equipped to fix everyone else's "boo-boos" too.
—*Mia Fraser*

Mom gives me a special drink every morning called NingXia Red (it sounds like Neeng-sha). It has orange and lemon essential oils in it.

I like to drink it plain, but Lisa likes to mix it with orange juice.

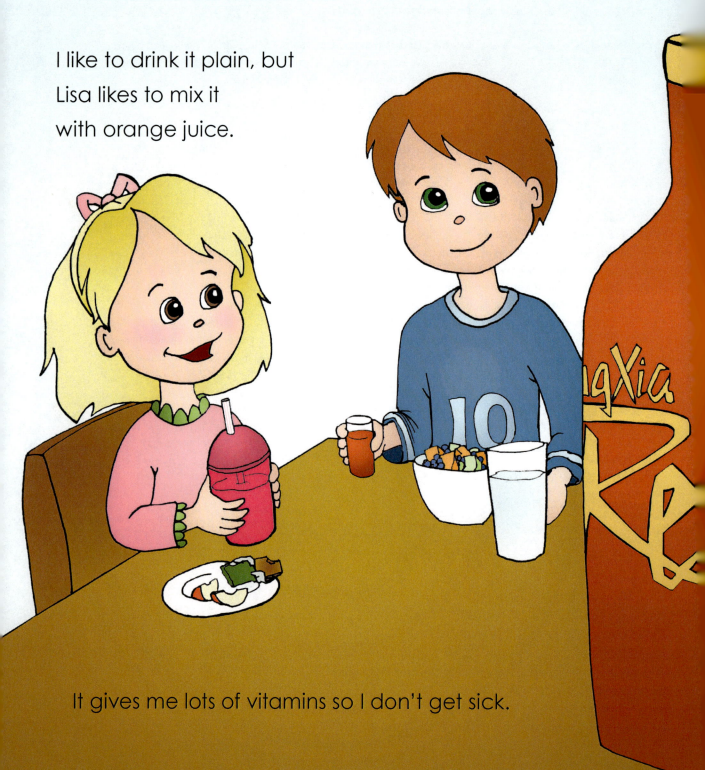

It gives me lots of vitamins so I don't get sick.

NingXia Red®

What is it? NingXia Red is a high antioxidant fruit puree made from the NingXia wolfberry, one of nature's superfoods. NingXia Red combines whole NingXia wolfberries with blueberry, pomegranate, apricot, and raspberry juices, and lemon and orange essential oils. It contains fiber, protein, and a variety of vitamins and minerals.[1]

How much can I drink? A serving size of NingXia Red is one ounce, although up to six ounces or more can be absorbed by the body. One ounce provides the antioxidant equivalent of the following entire list of foods: 4 pounds of carrots, 2 pounds of beets, 2 cups of beet juice, 3 cups of raspberries, 2 cups of blueberries, 2 quarts of carrot juice, 8 oranges, and 1 pint of orange juice.

How do I drink it? NingXia Red can be consumed straight, or it can be diluted with water or fruit juice.

What does it do for me? NingXia Red has been shown to be supportive of the immune and cardiovascular systems, and well as liver, eye, and cellular function. It is high in d-limonine, a powerful antioxidant, and wolfberry LBP polysaccharides have been shown to enhance the production of Interleukin-2 (IL-2), a cell protein that induces powerful cancer fighting responses.

Testimonials from Users

My husband and I use one ounce of NingXia Red daily and feel great. When we feel a cold coming on, we up our dose to two ounces for a couple of days and don't miss a step.

Our 8th grade daughter had a sore throat and felt a cold coming on. She took one ounce of NingXia Red for two days and was totally better. It was cute to listen to her passing on the advice to her six brothers and sisters.
—*Vicki Dau*

My 7-year-old daughter fractured her ankle and was put in a cast. About a week later she started really complaining of pain so after three days I took her back to the doctor. They took off her cast and found the cast had broken internally and was pushing into the back of her ankle. It was severly infected.

Her doctor prescribed a strong antibiotic and said they would have to have her come back in two days and possibly lance it. They were not even able to put a cast right back on because the infection was so severe they had to watch for blood poisoning.

I brought her home. Instead of filling the perscription, I covered the infection with Melrose®. I put Thieves®, Oregano, and PanAway® on the bottom of her foot. We gave her 4 ounces of NingXia Red. She went to sleep. When she woke up, the pain and infection were **gone**. I continued putting the oils on her for another week just to make sure everything was okay. We also kept her on the NingXia Red. She never had another flare-up.

When I took her to the doctor and told him what I had given her, he said I had been lucky she didn't end up in the hospital. And when they took repeat X-rays for her fracture they decided she didn't need another cast put on—after only one week with a cast on! The doctor told me sometimes "kids heal fast" … oh, okay!!
—*Shannon Hudson*

---

1. More information can be found at http://www.ningxiared.com.

We like to put lemon oil in our drinking water to make it taste good.

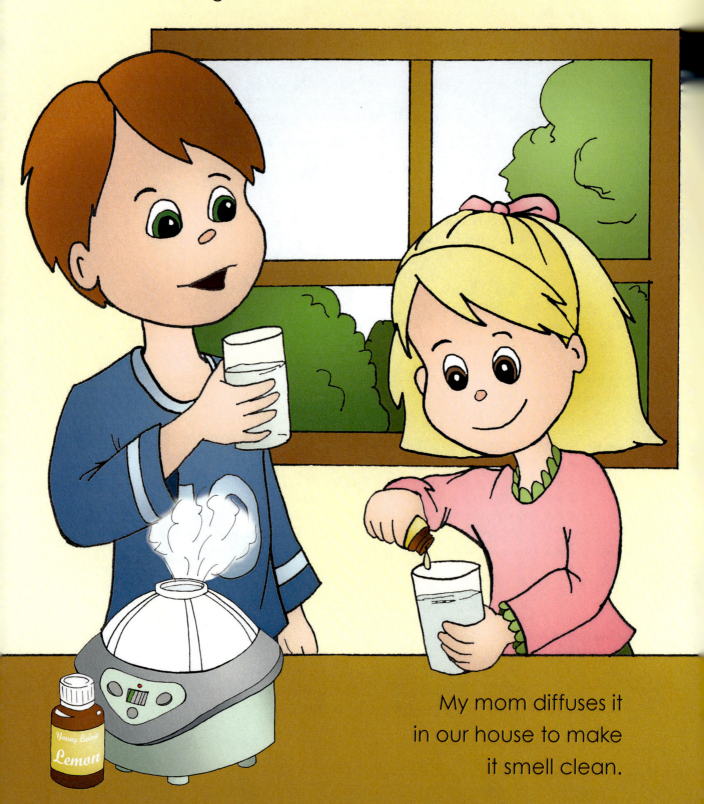

My mom diffuses it in our house to make it smell clean.

Lemon

What is it? Lemon oil is cold pressed from the rinds of organic lemons.

What do I use it for? Lemon has a fresh, clean, uplifting scent that has been shown to combat depression. It is antibacterial and can be used to help cleanse skin and combat irritations like acne and eczema. Lemon oil is high in the antioxidant d-limonine.

How do I use it?
- Apply directly on irritated skin (avoid direct sunlight for 12 hours after direct skin application, as citrus oils can cause sun sensitivity)
- Diffuse to clean and deodorize household air
- Apply to the bottoms of the feet to help fight infections
- Apply to the ears, diffuse, or directly inhale to combat depression
- Put a few drops in drinking water or on fresh or steamed vegetables to add a fresh lemon flavor
- Dilute with water and spray on fresh fruit to keep it from turning brown

Testimonials From Users

I know this sounds a wee bit out there, but my 19-month old granddaughter and the 20-month old girl next door like me to put lemon oil behind their ears and on their wrists when I do this to myself because we consider it to be perfume that smells pretty. Actually, I just adore the scent of lemon and since I knew this was healthy stuff, I didn't mind sharing one bit!
—*Marylou Cate*

Yesterday, my 3-year-old decided to take a permanent black marker to the new flat screen computer monitor we have. Trying to stay calm as I searched my brain for the right cleaner was a little difficult.

I put 4-5 drops of lemon essential oil on a tissue, and the marker wiped off better and more easily than a dry erase board! I was so suprised that I tried wiping it off without the lemon oil. That did absolutely nothing. I am so grateful for essential oils! There is no evidence left on the monitor except a nice smell!
—*Angela Geurts*

My 4-year-old got a wart on his hand from who knows where. We tried for several months with the over-the-counter stinky stuff. I then went to the expensive doctor that put more stuff on it that didn't work. Then I tried lemon oil. I put one drop on the wart two times and within a day it fell off. Why didn't I think of it a lot sooner?
—*Kimberly Reyes*

Thieves oil helps killl germs. My mom puts it in a spray bottle with water and sprays our hands and feet before and after school to help keep us from getting sick.

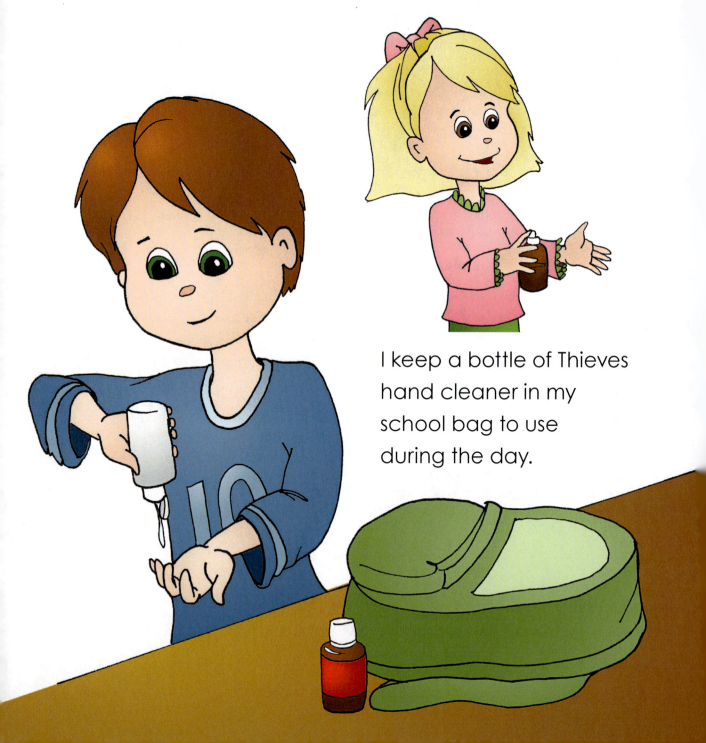

I keep a bottle of Thieves hand cleaner in my school bag to use during the day.

Thieves®

What is it? Thieves is a blend of essential oils that has highly antibacterial, antiviral, and antifungal properties. It is made up of clove, lemon, cinnamon bark, eucalyptus radiata, and rosemary oils.

What do I use it for? Thieves can be used to help combat bacterial and viral infections, including colds, sore throats, and fevers. It has also been shown to kill mold.

How do I use it?
- Diffuse Thieves to kill household germs
- Add 15-20 drops of Thieves to purified water in a 2-ounce spray bottle
    - Spray kids' hands and feet several times a day to promote immune function
    - Spray in the air to kill airborne viruses and bacteria
- Dilute with a carrier and apply to the bottoms of the feet, or the neck, chest, or spine to fight illnesses
- For sore throats, add a drop of Thieves to a glass of water; gargle and swallow (Thieves mouthwash is also great for this)
- Add a few drops to bath water to help combat illness

Young Living makes a variety of Thieves products, including toothpaste, mouthwash, dental floss, lozenges, bar soap, hand soap, waterless hand purifier, and household cleaner.

Testimonials From Users

Thieves is an oil that I *always* have on hand! When we go to public places where there a lot of other kids, I have my kids use Thieves on their hands to kill any unwanted germs. If anyone in our house is feeling under the weather, we load up on Thieves (on the bottom of their feet) to help boost their immune system.
—*Magan Weber*

The foaming soap is perfect for my young visitors who don't always wash their hands in the restroom as thoroughly as I might wish. Thieves takes care of that issue.
—*Marylou Cate*

My 8-month-old teething grandson recently came to live with us. I noticed him gnawing, chewing, and drooling at lot. I have a bottle of diluted (with V6 oil) Young Living Thieves blend that I keep on hand for rubbing my kids' (ages 4 and 7) feet. He was fussing so I tried one drop of the Thieves mixture on my finger then put it on his top and bottom gums. He was quickly happy and drooled a lot less. There was a delight-filled observation of the babies skeptical father! Now we grab the bottle of Thieves with the first sign of discomfort.
— *Sharon Lapierre*

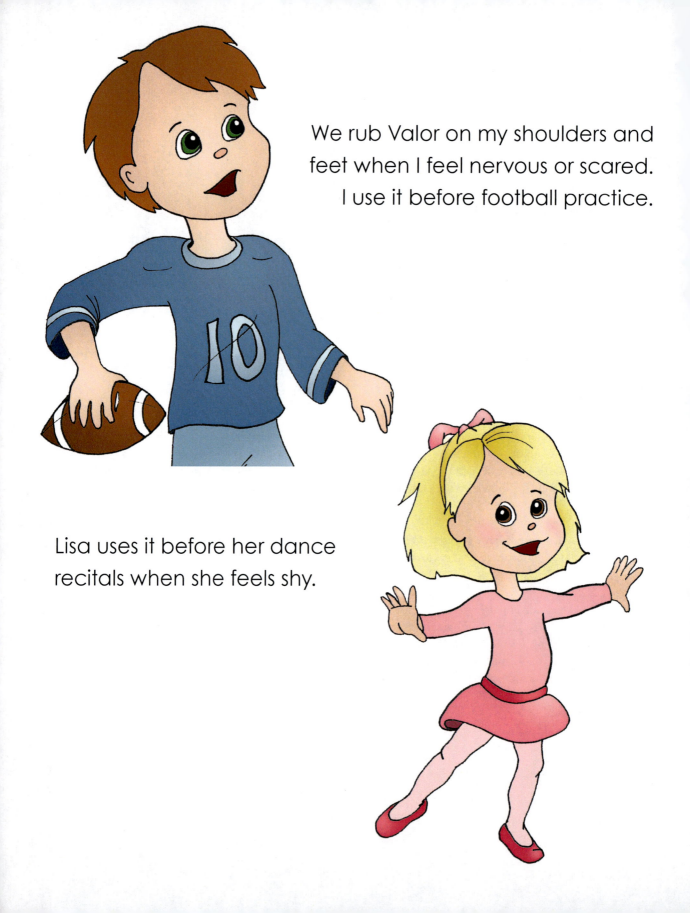

We rub Valor on my shoulders and feet when I feel nervous or scared. I use it before football practice.

Lisa uses it before her dance recitals when she feels shy.

Valor®

What is it? Valor is a blend of rosewood, blue tansy, frankincense, and spruce oils.

What do I use it for? Valor can be used to help promote confidence and self-esteem. It can combat nervousness and anxiety, and can help restore emotional and physical balance to the body. Valor may be useful in realignment of the spine.

How do I use it?
- Apply to the neck, shoulders, and bottoms of the feet to ease nervousness and promote confidence
- Apply along the neck, spine, and bottoms of the feet to help balance the body and align the spine

Testimonials From Users

My 12-year-old son tripped over on the concrete the other day before school. He came in and had grazed both knees and one of his elbows from the fall. He was visibly shaken, bleeding, and in pain.

I sat him down, added one drop of peppermint to each knee and the elbow and within a minute he said the pain was gone. He said his knees "felt creaky" so I added a drop of Valor to each knee (under the grazes). He then said "the creakiness" had gone too. I asked him how he was feeling, he said he was okay, then he proceeded to get ready for school, and walked to school!

There were solid scabs by the time he got home from school and I added another drop of peppermint to each of them, as he said they were a bit sore. Again, the pain was gone within one minute of applying. I didn't hear anything else about the grazes, except for a few days later when my son came in to show me how quickly they were healing—the scab had already started to come off!
—Jen Gallagher

When my daughter was in high school a few years ago she had some emotional problems, and as my first oil order I ordered a feelings kit. One day we went to a meeting where there were many people and she started panicking. About two weeks before, she had started this during school and it was creating problems with how people were reacting—teachers and students.

With my new kit in the car we left quickly and decided to pick an oil. I handed her the Valor essential oil and decided to have her smell it and put it on her neck. She immediatly calmed down and sat quietly for a few moments.

At the time when this had happened she had became more and more agitated and upset, but after the few moments she said, let's go back in, and I was amazed. Needless to say, I gave her a small bottle to carry with her and use as needed if she felt an attack coming on. Thanks to Valor and the other oils we used in the kit to work through some of the problems she was experiencing.

At this time, age 22, she doesn't need to carry Valor all the time, and for a long time she hasn't had a panic attack. I love the oils, the fact that they are natural and safe to use, and I'm thankful that they are so helpful for my family when we need some support.
—Karen Hammer

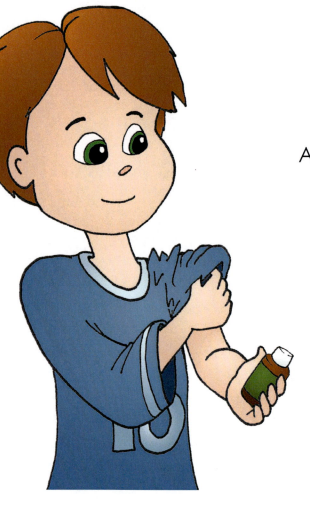

After practice, I like to rub peppermint oil on my sore muscles.

Lisa puts peppermint oil in a spray bottle and sprays herself to cool down after she dances.

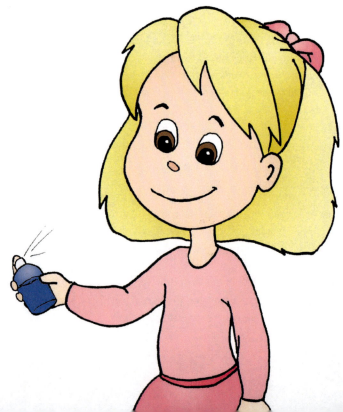

Peppermint

What is it? Peppermint oil is steam distilled from the mentha piperita species.

What do I use it for? Peppermint can aid in digestion and is antiinflammatory, antibacterial, and antiviral. It can also make a good pain reliever.

How do I use it?
- Apply 1-2 drops to the bottoms of the feet to help reduce fever (use a smaller amount for younger children)
- Add 10-15 drops to a 2-ounce spray bottle and spray for a cooling effect
- For digestive distrubance, put one drop in a large glass of water for drinking, or rub directly on the skin over the area of discomfort
- Apply directly to sore muscles or inflamed areas

Note: Peppermint oil should always be diluted with an organic carrier oil for small children or those with sensitive skin. It is best not to use peppermint oil on infants, as the scent can be overwhelming.

Testimonials From Users

I keep a bottle in my car to use when kid riders feel queasy on long rides. I also shared it with my pregnant daughters-in-law to help with nausea. Their doctors confirmed that essential oil of peppermint was a front-line defense for that situation.
—*Marylou Cate*

My 14-year-old son woke up at 3:30am one day with severe pain in his ear, side of his face, and throat. He had been having some sinus congestion prior to that, and I was suspecting that he may be getting an ear infection. Not wanting to go to an ER, I decided to use the oils again. This time I used lavender on a cotton ball, and placed it in each ear till morning. His temperature was up over 103°, so I also used peppermint (diluted, as it is too warm for my kids) on his chest and back.

He did get back to sleep, when before I could not even touch his face gently. When he woke three hours later, his pain was much decreased. We changed the cotton balls three times that day and continued with them in his ears. His temperature was down and he did not need further peppermint. By evening he was much better. All symptoms gone in a day and a half, with no recurrence.
—*Becky Lucas*

I use the oils all the time on my neices. Megan is 2½ years old and Courtney and Francesca are 5. Courtney and Megan love the oils and my sister-in-law *loves* that she no longer has to fight with her girls to take medicine! She uses the oils on them without hesitation, just in a smaller dose.

Francesca just started to let me put the oils on her this past Christmas. She was sick for Christmas and I told her she would be feeling better right away. I put peppermint oil (1 drop) on her chest and then a little V6 on top. Also, I put 1 drop in my palm, pressed my palms together, and rubbed them on the bottom of her feet. She was up and running around in half an hour. Now my sister is trying to implement the oils with her kids on a regular basis. The oils are perfect for children because no more trying to shove medicine down their throat and them spitting it out. Just a drop will do ya' on the bottom of the feet, and send them to bed.
— *Annamarie Desantis*

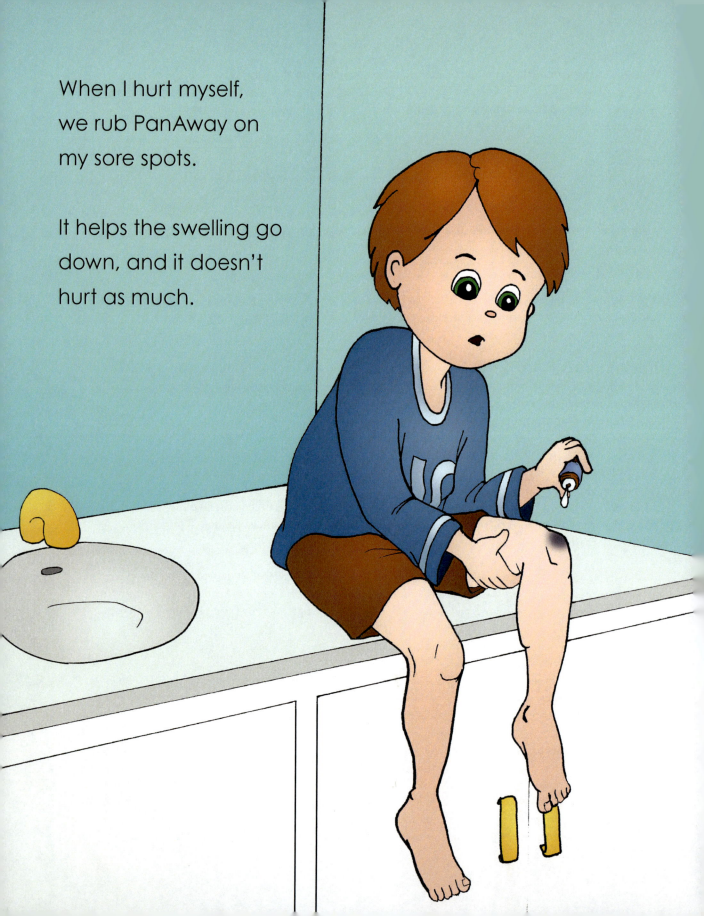

When I hurt myself, we rub PanAway on my sore spots.

It helps the swelling go down, and it doesn't hurt as much.

PanAway®

What is it? PanAway is a blend of helichrysum, wintergreen, clove, and peppermint oils.

What do I use it for? PanAway helps to reduce inflammation and aid in the healing of injuries. It can be used for strains, sprains, muscle pain, cramps, spasms, bruises, and deep tissue pain.

How do I use it?
- Apply PanAway directly to the injured area
- Use with a cold compress on injured tissue
- Massage into sore muscles or tense shoulders and cover with a warm compress

Testimonials From Users

My brother and his wife were visiting with their three children. The young one fell and scraped his knee. It was one of those abraisions with blood gushing, and looking a whole lot worse that it was. The parents moved into "Shall we take him to the hospital?" mode. He would not let anyone near him to wipe it to see what damage really had happened.

I reached for my PanAway, and asked him if I could just drop one or two drops of oil onto his knee assuring him it would not hurt. 30 seconds, perhaps 45 seconds later—wala!—he quit crying, he calmed down, and then said it didn't hurt too much any more.

Permission was granted to his parents to wipe away the dirt and gravel to see what the damage was. They wanted to get a band-aid, but he asked for another drop of oil, and after it was all cleaned he went back to playing. Life is much easier with kids when one has the Essential 7 Kit™ and especially PanAway.
—*Christine Carleton*

I use lavender oil when I get cuts and scrapes from football. They heal fast!

Lisa likes to mix lavender oil with lotion and rub it on her skin after she's been in the sun. Her skin feels better, and she smells good too!

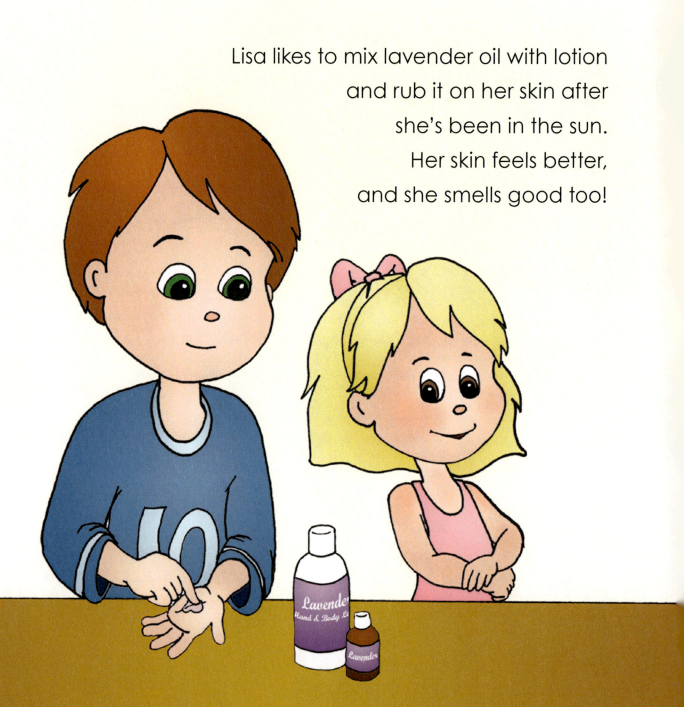

Lavender

What is it? Lavender oil is steam distilled from the lavendula angustifolia species of lavender flower.

What do I use it for? Lavender oil can help sooth skin irritations, such as cuts, scrapes, bruises, burns, sunburn, psoriasis, eczema, and acne, and can help prevent skin infections. It has been shown to help with both physical and mental relaxation.

How do I use it?
- Apply directly to skin irritations several times a day (dilute with an organic carrier oil or lotion on small children or those with sensitive skin)
- Apply to the neck, shoulders, or bottoms of the feet to aid in relaxation
- Diffuse to kill airborne germs and to aid in relaxation
- Add 3-10 drops to bath water before bedtime to calm children

Testimonials From Users

Lavender is the most used essential oil in our house. With kids, there are always an abundance, of bumps, bruises, scraps, and cuts, and lavender always soothes any "boo-boos" we have.

One morning my daughter awoke with a crusty, irritated eye. Throughout the day (4-6 times altogether) I rubbed some lavender on my hands and cupped it over her eye. Within 48 hours, her eye was completely back to normal.
—*Magan Weber*

What **not** to say about this *essential* essential oil? I travel with it to help me sleep (a few drops on the pillowcase helps when I am in a hotel) and I put it on my grand-girls' feet at bedtime after a light (no tickling allowed!) foot massage. Then I ask them to take a couple whiffs of my scented hands for good measure before tucking them in at night. My husband likes to use it on his pillow when he is fighting a cold. It helps him relax and sleep better.
—*Marylou Cate*

Lavender has been wonderful for my kids and their sore throats. A drop rubbed onto the front of the neck works, or, if they don't want to smell like the lavender, one drop in a small glass of water also works.
—*Becky Lucas*

I get a little paranoid when we get a notice from school that says someone in the class had lice. So I use lavender in the kids shampoo, and no worries for me! Never had a problem, and I feel better. I send them to school with a little plastic spritzer bottle in it with lavender, too, and they spray themselves down now and then.
—*Sondra Gerardi*

I like to diffuse frankincense when I do my homework. It helps me focus on my schoolwork and makes me feel happier.

Frankincense

What is it? Frankincense is steam distilled from the gum or resin of the boswellia carteri species.

What do I use it for? Frankincense is known as a "catch-all" oil and has an abundance of uses. It is immune supportive and has shown to be antiinflammatory, antidepressant, and antitumoral. It can foster positive attitudes and brighten spirits.

How do I use it?
- Rub on the neck, shoulders, and bottoms of the feet for immune support and relaxation
- Put drops on the ears and directly inhale or diffuse to combat depression or sadness
- Rub a few drops on the chest or spine to combat infections
- Put 3-10 drops in bath water to promote mental and physical wellness and relaxation

Testimonials From Users

If any of the kids is feeling under the weather, we give them a little modified Raindrop Treatment using frankincense and Thieves (and whatever other oils we might have on hand) with V6 oil (or other carrier oil) on their spine and back, and it seems to stop most illnesses before they barely get started.
—*Magan Weber*

My daughter had a wart on her leg and the dermatologist froze it off. It came back within a couple of months. We then tried a leading over-the-counter wart removal brand. It didn't go away. I finally remembered to check my essential oil book and found frankincense to remove warts. She started applying it two times per day, and within two weeks it was gone. It has been gone for over a year now and not come back. I have also had two other friends that have used it on their kids and it has removed their warts. Great stuff!
—*Cheri Moore*

For many years my beautiful daughter had struggled with depression. After taking prescription antidepressants for years, she had had enough with the pharmaceutical roller coaster. I suggested she attempt putting frankincense on the bottoms of her feet daily. She began doing that immediately and has been able to get off of all medications. She has now relied on frankincense alone for many months (6-7) and is feeling happier and healthier than ever before.
—*Carolyn Arkison*

When we play outside after dark, mom sprays us with Purification oil so we don't get bug bites.

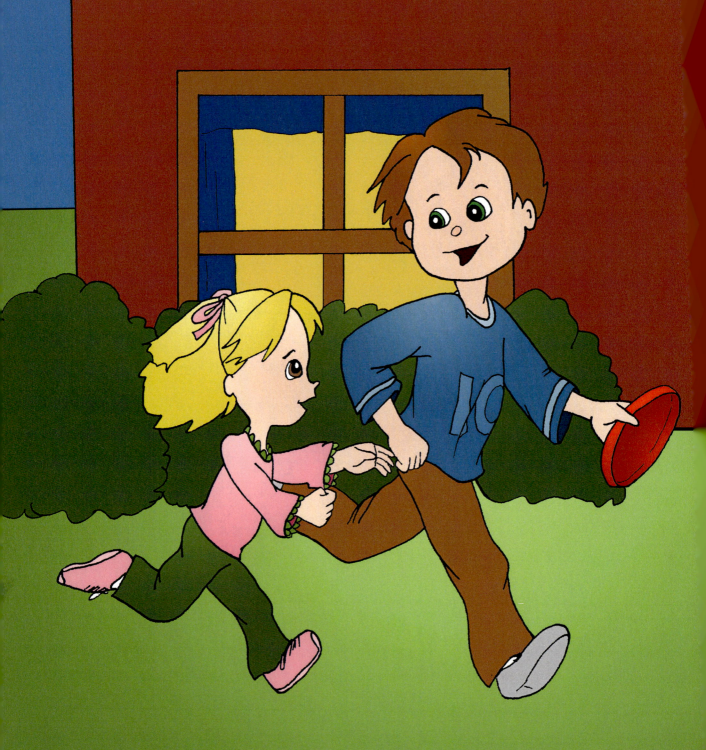

Purification®

What is it? Purification is a blend of citronella, lemongrass, lavandin, rosemary, melaleuca alternifolia, and myrtle oils.

What do I use it for? Purification cleanses and disinfects the air, neutralizes odors, cleanses skin, and can help prevent and heal bug bites and stings.

How do I use it?
- Put 20 drops of Purification in a 2-ounce spray bottle
    - Spray to disinfect the air
    - Spray on skin as a non-toxic insect relpellant
    - Spray on skin before swimming to inhibit chlorine absorbtion
- Apply directly to bug bites, scrapes, cuts, or blemishes to help them heal
- Diffuse to kill airborne germs and odors

Testimonials From Users

As a baby, my youngest daughter had lots of ear wax in her ears. After reading a testimonial online that said diffusing Purification helped rid a pet of dirty ears, I decided to try it for my daughter, and it worked great!
—*Magan Weber*

The summer my niece, Megan, was 3 years old, she was stung by something on her back left calf. Her calf was very red, hot, and swollen. You could even see the hole from the bite mark. Right away I grabbed my Purification oil and rubbed two drops over the area while her mom held her. Within 20 minutes, the swelling had gone down, and the redness and heat were gone. She was fine.
—*Annamarie DeSantis*

In the evening we use Peace and Calming oil to help us sleep.

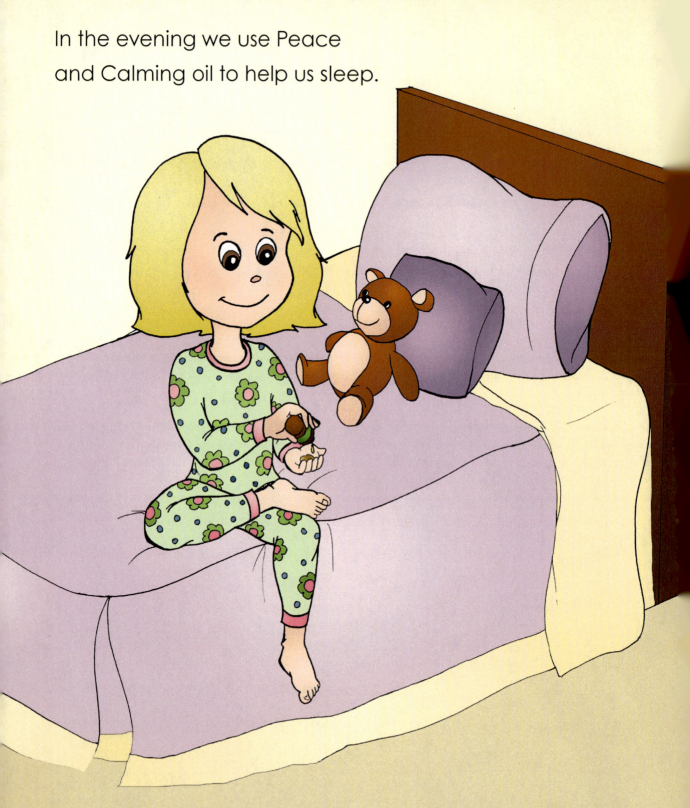

Lisa puts it on her feet before bed, and she sleeps well all night. She wakes up excited to use more oils!

Peace and Calming®

What is it? Peace and Calming is a blend of oils designed to promote peace and relaxation. It is made up of blue tansy, patchouli, tangerine, orange, and ylang ylang oils.

What do I use it for? Peace and Calming has an uplifting scent, and has been shown to reduce stress, depression, anxiety, and insomnia. It can help calm overactive children and promote sound, relaxing sleep.

How do I use it?
- Put a drop on children's feet before bedtime to help them sleep
- Diffuse to help calm children during the day or at night
- Massage on the neck and shoulders to calm stress or anxiety
- Add 3-10 drops to bath water before bedtime to calm children

Testimonials From Users

When my son was a baby, I would put Peace and Calming on my clothes when it was bedtime, so when I fed him and rocked him, he would fall fast asleep. Worked like a charm!
—*Magan Weber*

My brother and his wife and three kids were visiting and the first night the kids were pretty hyper. We rubbed Peace and Calming on the bottoms of their feet, and almost instantly they all calmed down and were in bed within about 15 minutes. My sister-in-law now uses either Peace and Calming or lavender on their feet just about every night before bed. Most nights she says they come to her and ask for their oils!
—*Vicky Goodridge*

I used Peace and Calming on my son, Tyler, as an infant when he was fussy and it seemed to help calm him down. I use lavender on the kids' cuts or bruises to help them heal. I use peppermint on myself whenever I get a tension headache which is usually a few times a month. It really does seem to help with the pain and makes the headache go away quickly.
—*Jessica Houston*

We love using Young Living oils in our house. They help make our lives happier and healthier!

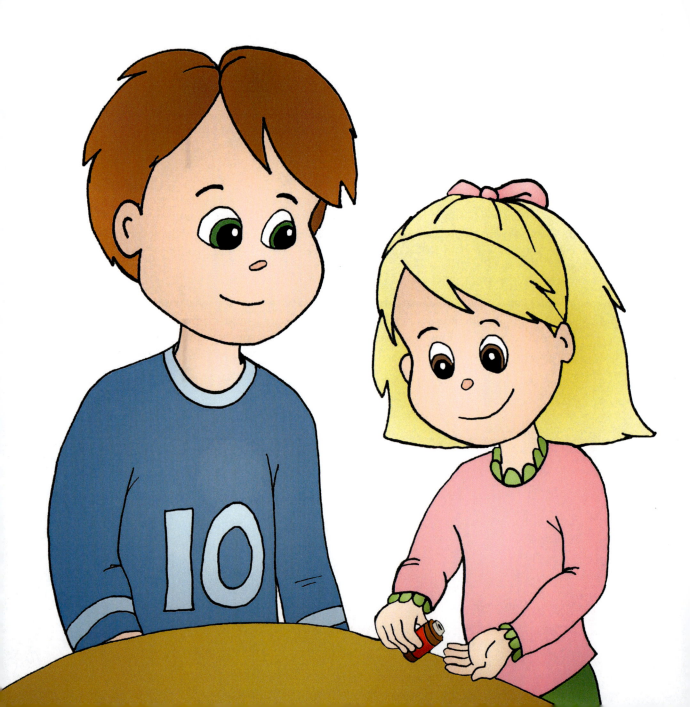

Child's Name _____

Oil Used	Condition	Amount Used	Application	Result

Parents: Use this table to keep track of which oils work best for your kids.

Records of Usage

Records of Usage

Child's Name _____

Oil Used	Condition	Amount Used	Application	Result

Parents: Use this table to keep track of which oils work best for your kids.